A Time for Healing

To Judith

With gratitude & best wishes,

Val H+W

by

Valerie A. Hodge-Williams

❁

photographs by Madelaine Gray

ISBN 0-935273-10

Published by CHESS Publications, Inc.
232 East University Parkway
Baltimore, MD 21218

Funding provided by:

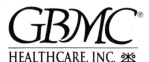

HEALTHCARE, INC. ❈

**The Greater Baltimore Medical Center
Comprehensive Breast Care Center**

This book is dedicated to the life and memory of

SALLY FISHER WILKES

A woman of rare courage and compassion

ABOUT THE AUTHOR

Valerie A. Hodge-Williams is a breast cancer survivor. She is also a licensed physical therapist who, prior to becoming a full-time writer, spent 27 years involved in direct patient care. The last 18 years of her physical therapy career were spent in home care and hospice, where her passion and specialty were focused on understanding and improving the recovery process of patients following catastrophic illness or trauma. During these years, her knowledge and expertise were greatly enhanced by her own personal experiences with major illness, including not only the breast cancer, but also a permanent brain injury and meningitis.

In addition to being a physical therapist, Ms. Hodge-Williams has a masters degree in adulthood and aging, with a specialization in suffering and survival. She is a board member of the Brain Injury Association of Maryland and a contributor to the organization's quarterly newsletter. She is also a frequent speaker on breast cancer, suffering and survival, and living with brain injury and chronic illness.

Ms. Hodge-Williams was born in Cheshire, England in 1948 and emigrated to the United States in 1973. She lives in the Baltimore, Maryland, area with her husband, John. They are the proud parents of three daughters.

❈

ABOUT THE PHOTOGRAPHER

Madelaine Gray is a professional photographer who has been selling her images for over ten years to publishing companies and at art shows. For many years she also worked as an occupational therapist, providing rehabilitation services in hospitals and out-patient clinics. Her love of art was stimulated by the art classes she took in college and at the New York Institute of Photography. Seven of her black and white photographs are on permanent display at Washington University in St. Louis. Her work is scheduled for group and solo exhibitions in 1998 in the Washington, DC metropolitan area.

TABLE OF CONTENTS

ACKNOWLEDGMENTS

My greatest gifts in life have come from the people surrounding me. Without the overwhelming, unconditional love of my family and friends, and the skillful and caring attention of the medical community, I would not have had the strength to fight my illness and write this book. There were many times when even an encouraging smile or a pat on the back meant the world to me, and I wish it were possible to acknowledge everyone who has enriched my life during my "time for healing."

I do, however, owe special debts of gratitude to certain specific individuals:

First of all, my deepest thanks go to John — my husband, lover, buddy, and best friend — for his unwavering love and support of me, for all his many and varied efforts on my behalf, and for his unfailing generosity and optimism. His presence at my side has been one of my most healing gifts. He is pure positive energy, and words could never express my debt to him.

The past years have not been easy on my daughters, Kelly, Erin, and Samantha. Yet, no matter how inconvenient or difficult were my problems or demands, they, like their father, never made me feel a burden. Instead, they showed me endless love, respect, and faith, often during times when I had none of these for myself. Their greatest gift of all to me was the way in which they used the entire experience to grow as individuals themselves. I could not be more proud or thankful for the strong and beautiful women they have become.

My sister-in-law, Maria Williams, fiercely believed in me as a person and writer despite our differing ideologies. My newly discovered siblings in Vancouver welcomed me with open hearts and minds. The initial contact with my sister, Catherine Holman, brother, Brian L. Mallard, and his wife, Sue Rigby-Mallard, only days prior to my diagnosis, was a great gift during a time that was otherwise full of loss.

My close friends Sarah Lazarus, Marte Herscy, and Lucy Ciesielski provided me with great relief during my recovery. Night after night over an entire year they listened to the "verse of the day" and gave me feedback and emotional sustenance. Anny Bakalian, another dear friend, read and edited my book at a time when my confidence in ever seeing my work in print was beginning to falter. Her enthusiasm gave me the boost I needed. Marty Lazarus and family, Marcie Weinstein, Bunny Murray, Patricia Mahone, Pat Cronin, Pat Hauptman, and Cynthia Ballard were always there for me when I needed them. The women with whom I worked out at the Towson YMCA gave me unfailing understanding, positive regard, and encouragement. My co-worker and friend, Mike Mauro, uncomplainingly assumed my physical therapy caseload, thus relieving me of worry. The generosity and commitment of these people and many others like them made even my darkest days bearable, and I shall always be grateful.

In the medical arena, Patti Wilcox, a Baltimore nurse-practitioner specializing in breast diseases, is a woman of rare spirit and also someone to whom I owe a very special debt of gratitude. Throughout the year that followed my diagnosis, she volunteered countless hours of her own time and expertise to give John and me much-needed guidance and invaluable advice.

Thank you also goes to the community and staff of the Greater Baltimore Medical Center for their excellent care of me throughout the years. I am grateful for the surgical skills of my doctors, Dr. Richard Hirata, surgical oncologist, and Dr. Bernard McGibbon, plastic surgeon, and for their wonderful care and compassion. Dr. Albert Blumberg, radiation oncologist, and the staff from "Special Imaging" — Pamela Murphy, Pamela Treat, and Madelaine How — unstintingly made time for me. They repeatedly reassured my fears and encouraged me to keep writing.

When the going got really tough, the positive regard and gentle wisdom of Dr. Irvin Cohen, psychiatrist, guided my mind through dark tunnels and out into the light.

Role models were essential to me, and I am very grateful for the courageous example of my quadriplegic cousin, Hazel Wilson. For me, she will always be the epitome of survival in the face of unending tragedy and loss. Nor will I forget the terrible suffering of my dearest cousin, Sylvia Billington. As I continue to grieve her loss, I am comforted by her memory and the message of her life. Sally Fisher Wilkes, to whom this book is dedicated, is another woman whose life I hold as a guiding light and whose death I will forever mourn. Sally's own terrible fight with breast cancer never diminished her zest for living, nor did it reduce her frequently superhuman efforts to help others who were also suffering. Thousands of us were touched by her short life.

I am also very appreciative of the invaluable lessons about suffering and survival that I received from the many patients I have treated over the years. They significantly enriched my understanding of illness, and I am grateful for their example and for the opportunity to share such an intimate part of their lives.

Last, but definitely not least, I thank all those who believed in the healing power of this book and made sure it was published. Betty Cox and Carole Hays of CHESS Publications, Inc., took an early interest as a labor of love. Madelaine Gray generously provided the beautiful photographs, bringing the verses to life. Brian Baker made the editing process a joyful adventure in learning. Linda Smeyne created an attractive package for the sample manuscripts. Dr. Alexander Munitz, radiologist, in his deep commitment to women's battles with breast cancer, read the manuscript and spent months searching for a sponsor. Without his vision and dedication, the book may never have come into being. My gratitude, delight, and surprise were complete when the Greater Baltimore Medical Center, the hospital that has so excellently cared for me and mine, agreed to fund the initial printing.

As I look back on the years since I wrote that first line, I realize that this book has come into being much like a quilt that has been stitched by many hands. Perhaps some patches are more noticeable than others, but the real beauty of the quilt is revealed only through the efforts and contributions of all.

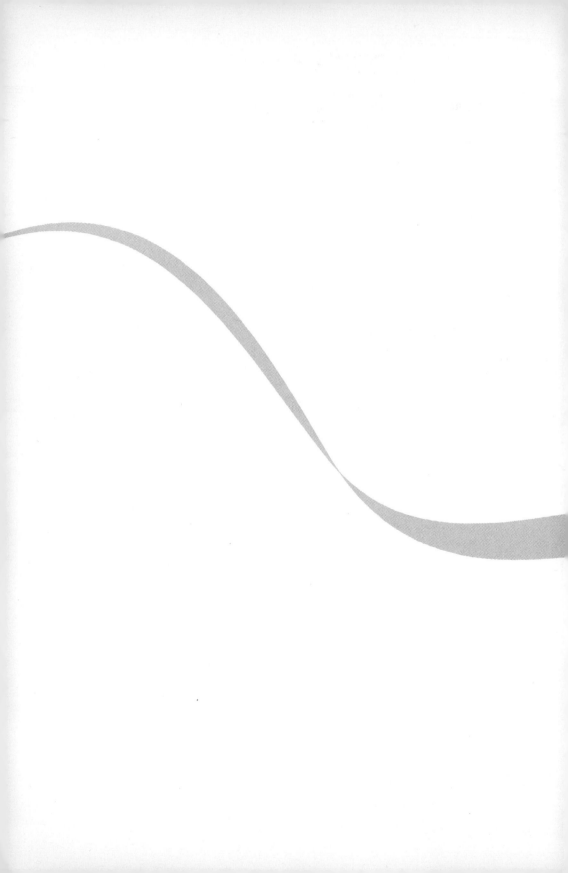

INTRODUCTION

It was a lump the size of a pea in the left breast. There was no sickness, no pain, no other symptom at all, just this pea-sized lump. A lump small enough to be missed and big enough to kill. Despite routine breast self-examinations, the discovery of this lump in my left breast was by accident. I was taking a shower and felt my hand rub over the lump's hard surface.

It always amazes me how the significance of time alters from one moment to the next. Usually, we live by quantifying these moments into minutes and hours. However, there are some that defy quantification. There is a timeless quality to them. They act as a boundary. Time thereafter is measured in terms of before or after that moment. Such was the significance for me of that moment in the shower. It altered my direction. In one instant, all the rules and expectations of my life changed, and I was forced into a turning I had not foreseen.

This was not my first experience with such moments. I had been involved with catastrophic sickness, in one form or another, since my early teens. My eighteen-year-old cousin, Hazel, had suffered a car accident that left her permanently paralyzed from the neck down. She and her mother had come to live with us following her discharge from the hospital. At the age of fourteen, without fully understanding it, I witnessed their amazing courage and determination as they battled through the feelings of a life forever altered.

Their journey had a lifelong impact on me: I chose to enter the profession of nursing and then the one of physical therapy. My progress in this field, however, was interrupted by another timeless moment: A head injury, at the age of twenty-three, left me with mild but permanent brain damage. One of the burdens from this damage was a diminished ability to administer physical therapy services in the clinic, due to the presence of too many concurrent stimuli. One of its gifts was that it forced me to search for other surroundings in which to practice. I began to specialize in home care and hospice.

In the patient's home, away from the sterile protection of the hospital environment, I found myself confronted by responses of both patient and family to the tragedy they had experienced. I became an uninvited witness to all of the feelings that illness and trauma evoke. Empathy became my greatest tool for both learning and treating. I soaked up the information provided by the patient, the family, and the home situation.

For those patients suffering from a terminal illness, stroke, or amputation, returning to a premorbid state was not an option. I began to redefine the term "healing" as a state of becoming, rather than one of returning. Yet I still did not have enough information to adequately assist my patients with the actual process. There appeared to be so much more to healing than the physical rehabilitation. I can vividly remember sitting next to a patient who had suffered an amputation. For no physical reason, he had stopped progressing. I thought "What is it? What essential piece of understanding am I missing?" Little did I realize at the time that I, myself, would soon be suffering from catastrophic illness and amputation. Within a month, I was diagnosed with breast cancer and underwent a mastectomy. In the year that followed, I discovered first hand many of those essential missing pieces.

When the cancer was first diagnosed, I used a strategy that had helped me to cope during times of stress in the past: I started to document my feelings in verse. What began as an individual journey of coping soon evolved into one designed to better understand and communicate the process of healing. I wanted to use the information to help others who were suffering, as well as myself.

I received overwhelming professional and personal support to continue in this effort of documentation. After one year, I had compiled a collection of sixty verses describing my process of healing. These simple poems lit my way through dark tunnels of shock, pain, reaching, ambivalence, tangents, and adaptation. Slowly and surely, they led me to the better lit paths of reintegration.

The patient in me discovered what the clinician could never have known: The feelings connected with the process of healing were very different from those of having healed. There were many times when I wished to deny the truth of those feelings. Irrationally, I felt guilty about acknowledging their intensity. The process of healing was sometimes shocking, even to me, in its raw admission of grief and pain. Only the encouragement surrounding me enabled me to stay true to the task. It compelled me to repress the urge to appear to be coping better than I really was and to document the truth of my experience.

Confusion was evident throughout the entire process. Often there would be a verse of hope, followed immediately by one of despair. Nonetheless, when all the verses were put into chronological order, the process flowed. As I reviewed each chapter, the faces of previous patients appeared before my mind, and I realized that even though some of the feelings were specific to breast cancer and some were specific to me, many of the verses could be generalized to illness and loss at large.

I never aimed to be a poet. The verses were written solely to document the feelings that occur during the healing process. Poetry was the only way I could express those feelings at that time. In the years since our battle with breast cancer, my family and I have been faced with many other timeless moments. Following each event, the process of healing has repeated itself, not necessarily in the same sequence. In these subsequent times, I did not need to write further verse. Even though the cause was different, my feelings were the same and had been already named. Many times, I would find myself repeating a verse from chapter 1, followed by one from chapter 5, then back to 3, and so on. Sometimes, I might only use four of the verses through the entire episode, but I would be comforted by them and would be able to move on.

I also used the verses to assist my patients. When they began to feel lost in their healing journey, I would ask them to choose a verse. It could be from any chapter, depending on where they were at that time in their process. Invariably, they would choose one describing anger or despair and find comfort in it.

I was not surprised by the positive response I received for these verses from the medical community and current breast cancer patients. The book had been written with both these populations in mind. However, I was surprised by the overwhelming support that I received from two other groups. In the first group were women who had undergone breast cancer some years back. The verses helped them to reexperience the recovery process in a safer time, thus gaining a form of closure. The second group consisted of the family members of breast cancer patients. The poems helped them to better understand their loved one's experience. Consequently, they were able to be more supportive during the process.

Many women are frequently reluctant to name the difficult feelings they experience as they endure their suffering from breast cancer. Sometimes, this is due to the coping method of denial, for which I have a healthy respect. Often, however, I believe it is due to the social taboo that appears to be attached to any answer other than, "Fine" to the question, "How are you?"

Difficult times are a part of life. Feeling awful and confused during them is appropriate. Naming the feelings helps to clarify the process. Admitting to painful and uncomfortable feelings is not a statement of giving up. It is a statement of courage, especially when the admission is accompanied by a struggle to continue the daily routine. The following verses can be read as a story, but more importantly, they can be used as a tool throughout these times of difficulty.

My message is one of hope. Do not confuse the process of healing with the experience of having healed. During the latter we feel successful and well; during the former it is appropriate to run the full gamut of bad feelings. Do not let them frighten you. Name them, express them, and move on to a better understanding and acceptance of life. Remember... nobody skips through suffering!

PART ONE:

MASTECTOMY

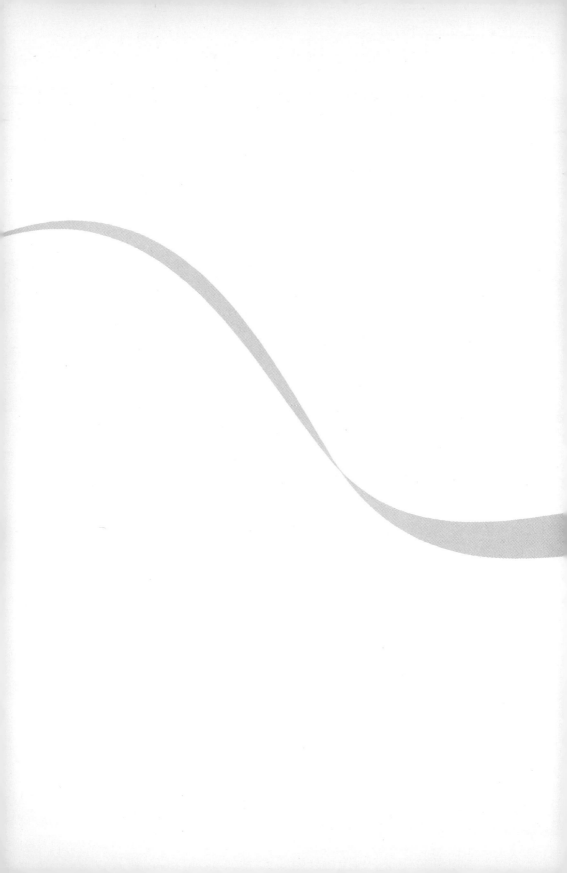

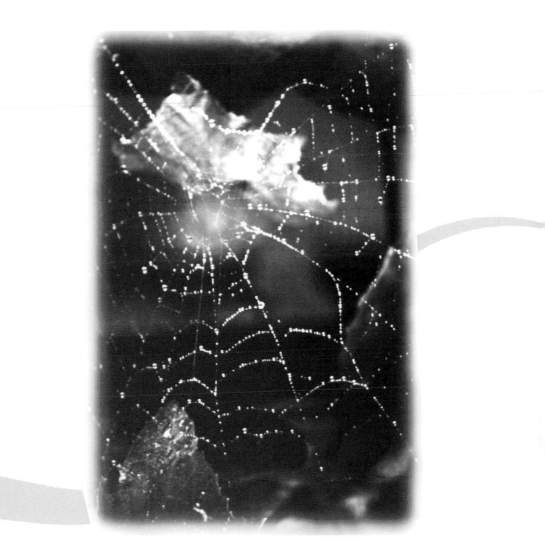

1 • A TIME FOR SHOCK

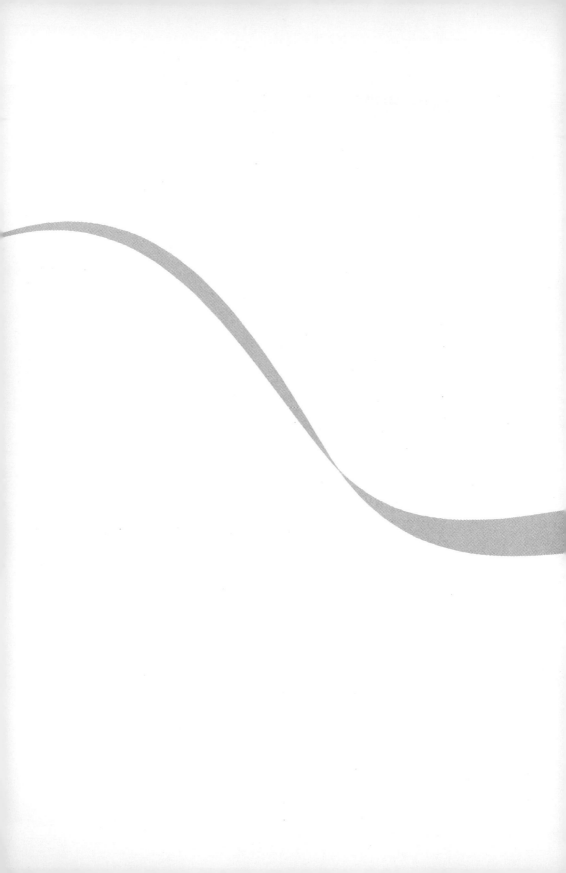

Wednesday, September 3

Yesterday, I went for a mammogram. The results were abnormal. Today, I am to make an appointment to have a biopsy. I feel split down the center. One part of me screams, "Danger!" The other shouts, "Impossible!"

TUMOR

I move through a mist on a web of silk strands
That quiver with each footstep I take.
I know they may hold 'til I reach the next shore,
And I know the next strand may just break.

No time since the start, no warning of voyage.
One day on a hill with a view,
The next in a mist with nothing secure,
Not even which thoughts to pursue.

As I stand on this web, I want to cry out.
To stand still 'til I gain back control,
To curl into a ball 'til a rescue is made
That will lift this deep dread from my soul.

I look at my mate on a web of his own,
Reflecting my fear in his eyes,
As he tries to reach out to support my next step
While attempting to muffle his cries.

And I know as I look that this is just life,
Not a thing on its own set apart.
And there's nothing to do but to trust the next strand,
In the hopes that the mist will soon part.

So I'll reach for my mate and we'll talk of our fears.
We'll cry for our loss of control.
We'll hold up our heads as we take the next step
And pretend we're just taking a stroll.

Wednesday, September 10

The biopsy was yesterday. It is now a fact. I have breast cancer.

QUEEN OF HEARTS

Off with your breast, now a cancerous growth.
Stop the disease at all costs.
Forget all the times that it's nurtured young heads.
Accept that the cause is now lost.

Don't think of your pride as a young woman grew,
In a bra newly fitted to breast.
Don't think of your mate and the passion that stirred
As your body was gently caressed.

It's time to forget all the good times before.
Think only in terms of your life.
Forget you were whole as you look at the odds.
Subject yourself to the sharp knife.

Come out of the sleep with a part of you gone.
Make sure that you mourn it with grace.
Don't hurt and don't care as you cast it away.
Prepare for the stares you will face.

Sunday, September 14

What a week. The doctor gave me a choice of treatment . . . lumptectomy with radiation versus mastectomy. Five days ago I knew nothing about either. Today I am almost an expert on both. I cannot seem to make the choice. I suppose I do not want to accept the need for it.

THE CHOICE

How did I get to this fork in the road?
How will I choose the best way?
Sharp rocks to the right, dark forest at left,
Through either I might go astray.

I'd like to turn back from this place where I stand,
Return to a landscape of green,
Where fields of wildflowers gave a scent of their own,
Where no hint of dark future was seen.

But there's no going back from this split in the path,
Not even much time left to stay.
I have to decide where to place my next step
And know no return from that way.

I look at the rocks and know they will cut.
I look at the trees with deep dread.
I stand at this place and cry out in vain
For the right not to walk, but be led.

I know this is wrong, not a way for my soul.
I'll not see if I hang down my head.
I must walk alone down the pathway I choose
And be sure of the ground that I tread.

For the rocks and the forest are not all that's there.
They're only what I can now see
From this place where I stand as the shadows of dusk
Obscure precious future from me.

There's a lot more ahead after forest and rocks,
Vast mountains and skies never seen,
Clear waters of streams and the colors of Fall,
Spring blossoms on trees budding green.

I'll force up my head to make the hard choice,
In the faith that the path I select
Is not there to hurt, but to lead me away
From this place that I cannot protect.

I stand now quite calm as the factors are weighed,
And each option's assessed with respect.
For I know without doubt that the progress I've made
Has come from the right to select.

Tuesday, September 16

The final pathology reports came back five days following the biopsy. They arrived as I was making the choice for lumptectomy with radiation. They proved the tumor to be five times greater than had been supposed and that there are two different types of cancer in the breast. All along, unknown to us all, my only option had been mastectomy.

PUCK

Waist deep in thick mud, all senses in fog,
Fierce terror attacking my soul,
Frozen in fear, numb and in shock,
How did I fall down this dark hole?

I was walking a path in the twilight of day.
At the fork of two roads I'd been strong.
With my head held up high, I was ready to move
When Fate's Fool showed my choice to be wrong.

Oh, he laughed at my shock, yes, he howled with great mirth,
Held both his sides from the pain.
As he jeered at my plight, he perceived with delight,
All my faith in the choice was in vain.

And I fell, as I heard his false echoes of words,
Into this hole dank with mire.
As I face now with pain the hard rules of the game,
I refuse at this time to retire.

I'll thumb up my nose at this jester of fate,
Throw back his loud cackles and cope,
Reduce him in size, as I prove to his eyes,
I still have my faith, strength, and hope.

Once more on the road, after clambering out
From this pit that I hadn't foreseen,
I note with wry wit that although I'm quite fit,
Each day I'm a little less clean!

Thursday, September 18

I was told I could have the option of breast reconstruction at the time of mastectomy. Unfortunately, no plastic surgeon had any operating time available. In desperation, I accepted my only alternative, a seven o'clock in the morning appointment for consultation.

GLIMPSES BEYOND

Nine days have now passed since the biopsy's truth.
The mastectomy's scheduled tomorrow.
I'm trying to maintain a stiff upper lip,
But my soul is immersed in its sorrow.

Time has flown by in a flurry of tests.
I've researched and heard everyone's voice.
Though it's helped me stand firm through this hurricane time,
In review, I've been left with no choice.

In another bland office I wait without hope
For a skilled plastic surgeon, who'll state,
"I'm sorry, tomorrow my schedule's complete.
Therefore, your reconstruction must wait."

I'm unsure why I've come, since I know his techniques
Must give time for the sutures to heal.
What's the point until then in discussing effects
Which his artistic knives will reveal?

A film's shown, as I sit, which begins to explore
Three options by which a new breast
May be formed from the tissues of tummy or back
Or by stretching the skin of the chest.

It's again more to learn, overwhelming right now.
I can't see through the dread of tomorrow,
But the surgeon arrives, and his gentle intent
Begins lifting my burden of sorrow.

As he shows me some slides of the women he's helped
And explains all procedures in full,
Hope pierces the depths of my darkest despair,
And the edge of my pain starts to dull.

My ordeal is now faced with a spirit renewed,
Though tomorrow still comes bringing grief.
I've been made aware, in a beautiful way,
Reconstruction can offer relief.

Friday, September 19

    D day. Everything is in order. This is the time I have been dreading. After today there will be no looking back. My journey to the hospital is only the first step. God give me the courage to take it!

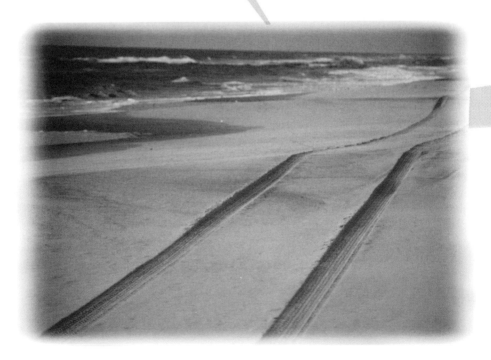

DEADLINE

An overcast day, move slow in a trance.
Perform all your actions by rote.
Focus all strength on the journey ahead.
In three hours you'll be able to float.

Channel all thoughts from the loss of this day.
Think not of pain, nor of grief.
Think only of love as you start on your way,
And know the next step will be brief.

You just have to get to the hospital doors.
Take a hot shower, clean your teeth.
Choose all your clothes with unusual care.
Don't let your strong guard know relief.

Say "Bye" to the girls and hug them with love.
Give them your thanks for the way
They've given their support throughout the past weeks.
They'll see you at close of the day.

Look to your love and his strong gentle face.
Think of his care and his touch.
Try to express what his presence has meant,
But know there's no words for how much.

Time to get up, to move on your way.
Time to leave children and mate.
Time for the start of your journey alone,
But know they will lovingly wait.

Into the car for the final few steps.
Hope you have all that you need.
Time to let go of the fight to control.
Time now for others to lead.

Again in admissions, the butterflies start.
Battle them back with all force.
Calm down "fight and flight," calm down as you write.
Let the day take its predestined course.

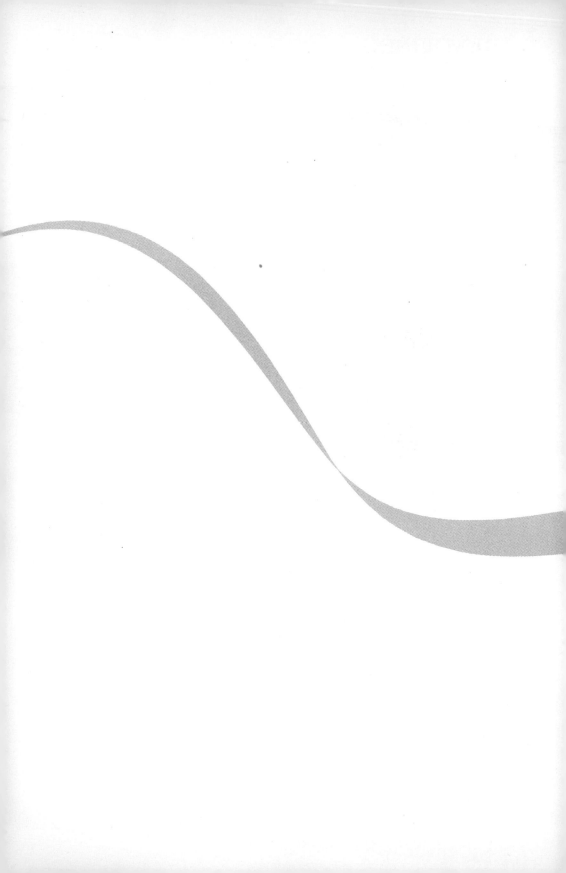

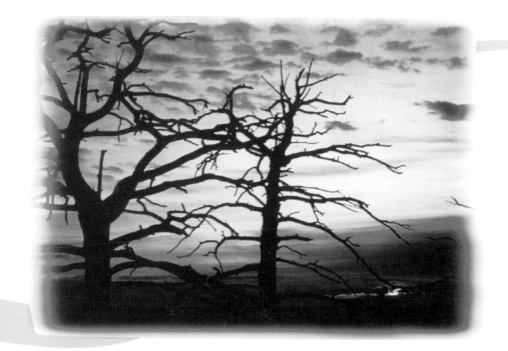

2 • A TIME FOR PAIN

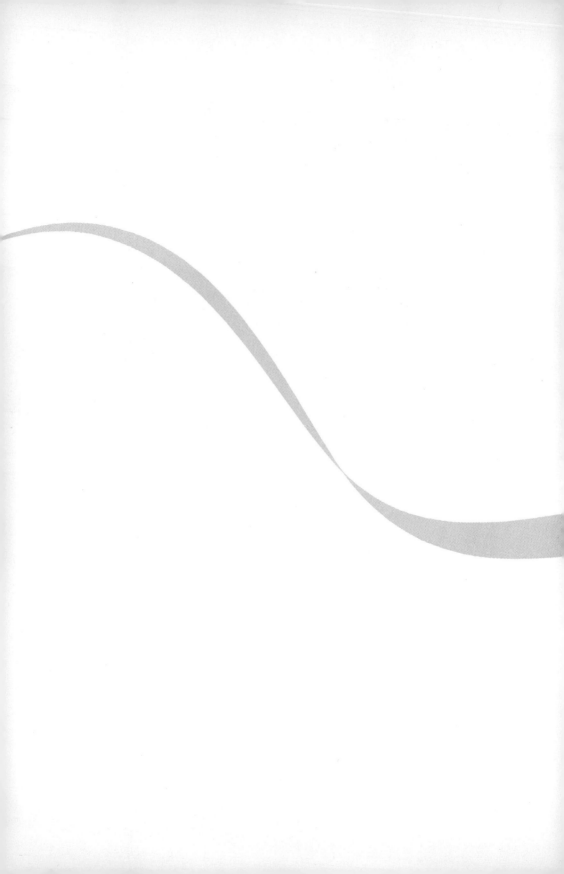

Sunday, September 21

   3 am. . . . I have been lying awake for hours.
My postsurgical time has proceeded without
complication. Now, without warning, my
euphoria has disappeared, and the fantasy has
cracked wide open.

GOBLINS OF THE NIGHT

Pain and horror, loss and grief, screaming in my soul.
Tubes and staples in my side that close a gaping hole.
Panic racing through my heart, which beckons "fight and flight."
These old fiends I've seen before, they're Goblins of the Night.

They visit as I close my eyes. They banish hope of sleep.
They laugh and jeer and terrify me as I softly weep.
They whisper that one breast has gone and cancer's lurking near
To take my other breast away, perhaps my life next year.

The panic starts to reach a pitch I cannot bear alone.
I'm frozen in what next to do, as I don't wish to phone
My loved one, who so needs his sleep and time away from grief.
I call the nurse without much faith that she can bring relief.

I hate to ask for medicines. I'm worried that they'll take
My independence from this fight and only serve to make
The grieving period longer, therefore harder overall.
But now I'll grasp at anything to make the Goblins fall.

I slowly drift away with peace into the dark of night.
From fears and terror I have found a drug-induced respite.
I need to know, within my soul, when is the time to fight,
And when's the time to ask for help 'gainst Goblins of the Night.

Tuesday, September 23

The house doctors are uncomfortable with my grief. I must be in a very fragile time to be so upset by this. I seem to need all of the reassurance I can get.

THE HEALER'S GIFT

Young man, do you care?
Are you threatened by my pain,
Or don't you even let it get that near?

Young man, are you wary of my need?
What can it do to you?
I feel your blocks against me!

Young man, I see you want to try.
A dream is in your eyes.
Are you frightened of exploring uncharted territories?

Don't you know it takes more than books
Or a stethoscope around your neck
To be a healer?

Did you think you could heal bodies
Without touching souls and minds,
And remain untouched yourself?

Did you think you could meet with pain and death
And remain unchanged?
Is it the intimacy you fear or the helplessness?

Human frailty has always been a constant.
Failure exists only...
If you turn away!

Young man, don't waste the dream.
Share the intimacy of suffering, pain, and loss,
And the gift will grow!

Thursday, September 25

I am due to go home tomorrow. I am just
waiting for them to remove one of the drains.

THE FACADE

"Are you ready?" he asks, as I open my eyes
And sleepily focus on his.
I'm not sure what he means, but can sense a surprise
That perhaps I would rather just miss.

A month of hard shocks since the dread lump's arrival.
A month of fear, pain, loss, and grief.
Enough now! I've paid the high price of survival.
I've had it! It's time for relief!

But no, here they stand 'round my hospital bed,
Bright, healthy, and smart in white coats.
I note, through their charm, that their purpose today
Involves more than to look or take notes.

My fears are allayed as I find with relief,
They intend to remove the front drain.
I'm glad of this fact, since it's been in the way
When I move, often causing me pain.

One takes out a stitch, another looks on.
I relax and then tense with a shout.
The sensation I feel is my breast torn away
As six inches of tube is ripped out.

It's not that they're cruel, nor the pain so severe,
That causes this level of shock.
But the physical tear of that drain from my wound
Makes firm doors of denial unlock.

A week has now passed since my surgical loss.
'Though I slept as they took it away,
I've massaged the scar and I've looked in the glass,
But have fought off the truth 'til today.

It's been fully unveiled by the rip of that drain.
I now know it was more than a dream.
The facade is collapsed, as deep vulnerable rage
Floods with grief, through my soul, on a scream.

Sunday, September 28

I am home at last! John, my husband, has
been so loving and supportive throughout this
time, I wonder what he is really feeling.

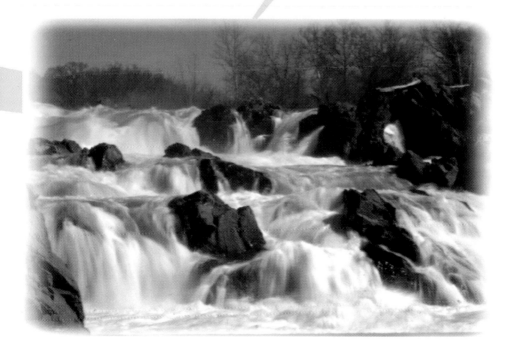

TOGETHER ALONE

My eyes reach for his.
Can we pass this test?
Will I see his disgust
Or mine?
Or will he protect me
From both?
How will I feel?
How will he?
I am no longer the same.
I look down.
I am nine years old....
    I have not seen
That left side from this height
    since then.
It is not repulsive
But strange.
I look different.
Another person on one side,
My old familiar me on the other.
A man from the left,
A woman from the right.
Which am I?

My eyes reach for his.
Tears fall.
His and mine.
No longer whole,
No longer worthy.
He cries not for my loss,
But for his inability
To protect me from it.
His fault!
His role was to protect.
My fault!
My role was to be perfect.
We cry together for
    our foolishness,
And then we face
What we have refused
    to acknowledge...
The cancer!

It was cut out.
It had to be.
I hurt, he hurts,
It had to be.
No one's fault,
...It just had to be.

Monday, October 6

My Achilles' heel was always my bladder. I have now developed a urinary tract infection as a side effect of the past month's stress. On some level, I do not seem to be able to believe all of this is really happening to me. Irrationally, I feel as if I must have done something terrible to deserve it.

THE GIFT OF FALL

Surrounded by the flowers of Fall,
My spirit drifts inert.
Melancholy pervades my soul,
Too worn to even hurt.

The season meets my mood of loss,
Though not, it seems, my grief.
For colors shout from every flower
And every golden leaf.

I note that Summer's come and gone.
Now Autumn's passing too,
And Nature wants to celebrate
With shades of every hue.

A paradox it seems to me,
That dying things should blaze
With such accepting beauty,
Through their final Autumn days.

I lie here sore and listless.
My anger shouts, "Why me?"
I'm mad at every lovely flower
And every golden tree!

How can they take so peacefully
What I with rage resent,
That there are things within this life
That nothing can prevent.

The trees and flowers appear empowered
By Nature's sense sublime
To give each minute its own worth
And all things their own time.

So why can't I, in my despair,
Accede to Nature's way,
Accept with grace the loss and pain
That is my path today?

Perhaps Fall in her glory
Not death alone does sing,
But heralds Winter's coming,
Which, in turn, gives rise to Spring.

Hence, may each different season
And each phase of life within
Rejoice both in the moment
And in what its loss may win?

Thus drifting through the flowers of Fall,
In Nature's faith I find
A key to free my wounded soul
And heal my tortured mind.

I'm just a part of Nature's force,
My breast a part of me.
I'm special as each lovely flower
And every golden tree.

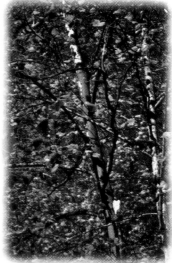

And when their stems begin to droop
And leaves begin to fall,
I'll share their loss and know with grief,
It's common to us all.

Therefore, I'll try to live my life,
However long it be,
With Nature's joy in every flower
And every golden tree.

Friday, October 10

All day I have been in the thrall of pending doom. I keep trying to think away from it. I am frightened that it will disintegrate the positive attitude that I am so desperately trying to achieve.

DEADLY GAME

There is a screaming deep inside
I dare not go too near.
It's very vague, but it portrays
The essence of my fear.

There is a shade that stands up close
Which I don't dare to see.
I quickly look the other way
In case it comes for me.

There is a sound which fills my ears
That I don't dare to hear.
It's calling names all indistinct,
I dread mine will be clear.

There is a touch I dare not feel,
Nor taste, nor smell the same.
For should I dare to do these things,
Then Death may win its game.

Saturday, October 11

    I have been shouting at the children again.
My teeth are so on edge, I could scream!

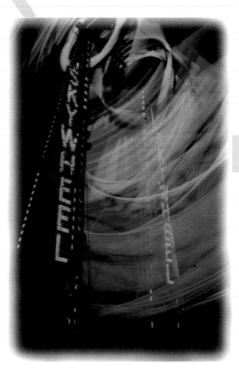

MOOD SWINGS

One day I write of faith and hope,
The joys I take in Fall.
The next it's of despair and rage
And fears that death will call.

One minute I'm so full of life,
I'm champing at the bit.
The next I feel so worn and tired,
I'll never more be fit.

One hour I'm sure I'm beautiful,
Despite the breast I've lost.
The next I feel my life was bought...
My youth and looks...the cost!

One moment all my children,
My mate, and friends I need.
The next I scream to be alone,
From people's presence freed.

One second I'm so normal,
The old me from before.
The next I'm strange and different,
A freak forevermore.

They say in all the literature
That moods may tend to swing,
But they omit to mention
The chaos these moods bring.

How can my loving family
And faithful friends succeed
To give the help they wish to give
If I don't know my need?

I'm tired of all these ups and downs,
Of swings I would be free;
But most of all, in all this fuss,
I'm bored with being me!

Sunday, October 12

My days are all merging into one. I never knew that heavy self-preoccupation could be so boring.

HUMOR

It's time, I think, for lighter verse
Amidst this doom and gloom.
For even through these stressful times,
For humor there's been room.

We found it stashed in places where
We'd no intent to play,
For instance, the recovery room
Where many hours I lay.

They asked me if I'd give my name.
To test my mind they tried.
I knew, but found the query rude,
So with intent I lied.

They asked me then how old I was.
I'd lost that little key.
I tossed some numbers 'round my head
And chose a twenty-three.

Take heed from this, you cannot win.
Note what they did to me.
They kept me there for ten whole hours,
Without one cup of tea.

The next event that I recall,
With humor more bizarre,
Was when my loved one and myself
First looked upon my scar.

We faced the glass both faint of heart,
Unsure that we could rise
With courage to this greatest test,
Afraid we'd hide our eyes.

To our delight, we both beheld
(With some denial I fear)
A tattooed female warrior's form
That only lacked a spear!

From this we gained a cherished time,
Adjoined forever after
By changing that potential shock
To helpless healing laughter.

The bra came next with puffed-up breast
To my dear husband's glee,
Who found he'd swapped a thirty-four
For forty-two, size D.

We howled with mirth, I do recall,
When this first bra I tried,
For now my form appeared as if
I'd lost the other side.

Amidst these reminiscences
I've, with surprise, revealed
How much throughout these darkest times
The power of laughter healed.

Although my verse at first began
With attitudes quite flip,
I now perceive in each event
A most important tip:

To all times there's a funny side.
With humor, great relief
Is found, if one can bear to search
Through suffering, loss, and grief.

Wednesday morning, October 15

The last drain is out. I am frozen in panic. I never realized how much that tube in my side had prevented the redefinition of my new body limits. I am lopsided and off balance. My soul has no place for this new shape. It keeps searching for its old one!

JOURNEY ALONE

Go away! Leave me alone!
I'm frightened this grief will scare you
The way it scares me.

Let me hurt now in peace,
Without facing inquiries
Into my health.

Let me scream on my own.
No more trying to maintain
A brave front.

I'm sick of the people
With stupid remarks
Without thought.

They're sure I'll be fine.
What do they know?
I'm not fine.

They infer
They'd be fine.
They wouldn't.

I must live for today.
Can't they see? Are they blind?
It's today I can't bear.

Let me cry,
Please let me cry,
Let me rage.

I'd like to smash windows with bricks,
But they'd put me away
In a room with some pills.

So leave me alone.
Let me scream, please,
In peace!

Wednesday afternoon, October 15

Everyone agrees on the importance of a positive attitude, but they all vary on its description. After these past six weeks, I think I can describe it very accurately in one word... ELUSIVE!!

A GOOD ATTITUDE

The doctors all say,
"A good attitude counts."
Does this mean
Don't think about
Cancer or death?
Well, I have,
And I'm frightened by both!

The doctors all say,
"A good attitude counts."
Like saying
"Learn English
In France,
 Without teachers or books."
A statement, no more.

A cancer has struck.
I've lost my left breast.
My faith in this body
Is under attack.
I'm in physical pain
And emotional grief.
But since they all say,
"A good attitude counts,"...
I'd like one!!

Friday, October 17

It has been four weeks since the surgery. The drain is out and the wound is healed. It is time to move on. At the start of the month, I had fantasized a brilliant recovery. It didn't work that way. Instead, I learnt a little more about human frailty. I suffered, raged, feared, and was loved. Most important of all, I survived.

FEELINGS

Grief is so lonely.
I'd not understood this before.
It can never be shared.
It's unique to the intimate core
Of us all.

Rage overwhelms
With its threats to take over control.
It distances others,
Who sense its repression and fear a response
From their soul.

Fear is so dark,
With its boundaries vague and unclear.
It has to be fought,
Or it tends to consume all the positive thoughts
That come near.

Love is so warm.
It expands and breathes life with its touch.
It can always be shared,
And its gift during grief, rage, or fear
Can ease much.

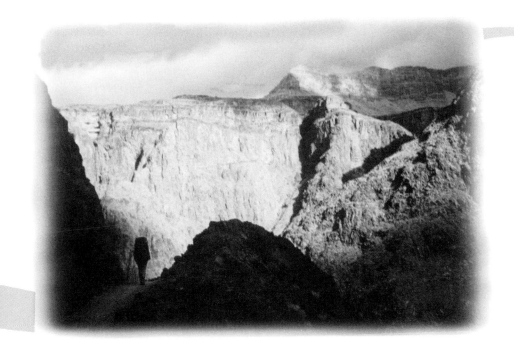

3 • A TIME FOR REACHING

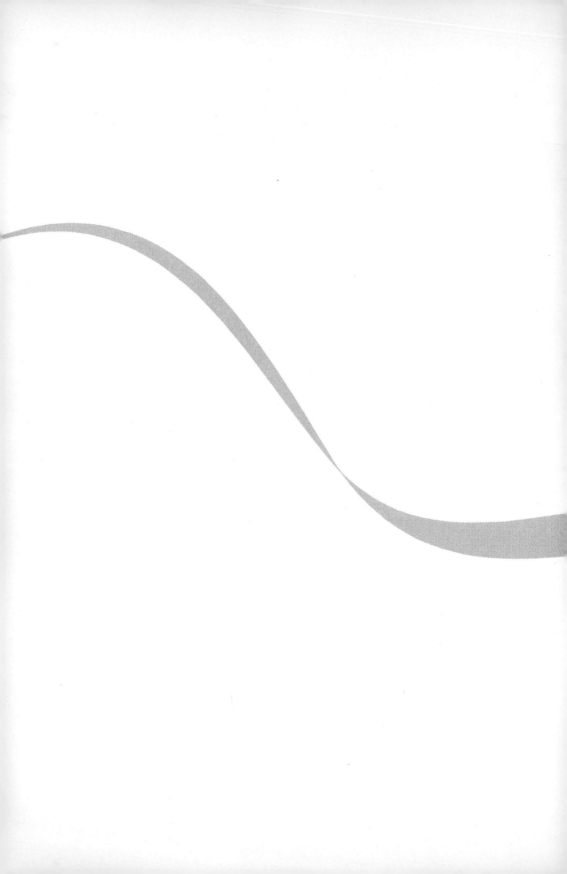

Sunday, October 19

This is a difficult time. I am so unsure of myself. Everything feels new.

FIRSTS

First time in the shower
With no tube in my side
For the drain.

First feelings of freedom
In washing myself
Without pain.

First heart-stopping shock
    as I wash
The right breast and then reach
For the left.

First anguish from functions
That show in what way
I'm bereft.

First venturing into
The crowd with a
Temporary breast.

First fears it's lopsided,
Or shaped wrong, to pass
The symmetry test.

First dread as I see
My reflection in
Altered swimwear.

First cringing of soul,
    as the scar
Shows the world what is
No longer there.

First intrepid doubts that my
Loving will fail in my
Lover's embrace.

First sharing of tears as I
Nakedly turn
And him face.

First knowledge of space
That I no longer fill
Quite the same.

First raging and
Grief-stricken battles with
Feelings of shame.

First vexing by clichés
From folk who don't know
    there is
Nothing to say.

First heart-giving thanks
    for the friends
Who've shared love in their own
Special way.

First faltering steps
In a world that is
Changed evermore.

First sighs of relief as these
Steps start becoming
Increasingly sure.

First success as a night
Without nightmares gives way
To a dawn.

First glimmers of faith . . .
Life continues despite
What we mourn.

48

Wednesday, October 22

I have an appointment with the surgical oncologist this afternoon. I am looking forward to showing him my progress. I am trying to ignore my other reality, which is that he may find more cancer.

THE WAITING ROOM

I sit in the waiting room,
Looking at others who are
Waiting, like me.

We all have one aim,
Though a different approach:
To live longer in health.

No one talks, no one laughs.
A silence pervades.
Is it fear?

I notice the Specters of Cancer and Death
Sitting near to
Each person.

That's why we are here.
Let's not give them more power
Than they already have.

We each wait for our personal sentence.
Could it be freedom?
Probably not.

So why do we choose to allow
Isolation to breed, as we sit here and wait
In this room?

I'd like to reach out
To the others
And say,

"I know what it's like.

I know you know, too.

And I'm sorry!"

Friday, October 24

Routine physical examinations are no longer boring!

THE EXAMINATION ROOM

Shock, confusion, darkest fear,
Freezing souls where they appear,
Nameless terror in their breath,
Ghostly specters...Cancer! Death!

Killing peace, dispelling hope,
Squashing fight and skills that cope,
Screaming horror as they loom
In each examination room!

I've come, at last, to know their game.
Their power is in my fear to name
Their presence in my everyday,
My need to look the other way!

It's now the time for me to face
My constant fear of their embrace,
Refute the lying doubts that say,
"Ignore them and they'll go away."

At first I'll try accepting fate.
Then Cancer's threats I'll integrate.
Determined in this fight to win,
But still unsure how I'll begin.

Their greatest strength is unnamed fear.
I'll stand my ground when this comes near.
I'll name it loud, with head held high,
And thus both specters I'll defy.

It may take time to win this fight.
But one day soon, I'll earn the right
To send them packing if they dare
To threaten me. So...GHOSTS BEWARE!!

Saturday, October 25

I am sick and tired of the philosophies of suffering. When I have asked others how I will cope without nipple sensation, they tell me that everything will be fine, and I will develop other sensitive areas. But what do I do in the meantime? Every time we make love, I am made aware of my loss at its deepest level. The grief becomes so overpowering that I want to run from all intimacy.

ALTERED LOVING

From the deepest of my dreams
To his loving touch I waken.
Gentle stroking.

In the safety of his arms
A warm embrace is given.
Passion mounting.

In the stillness of the night
A rising flame's extinguished.
Something missing.

From the site of amputation
There is lack of stimulation.
Silent screaming.

By my body is demanded
A sensation lost forever.
Altered loving.

Sunday, October 26

I have been forcing myself through lovemaking. I know that I haven't fooled my husband, John, for he senses my grief. Neither of us knows what to do. We are trying to continue as if things were normal, in the hope they will soon improve. He must be as frightened as I am.

JOHN

You were there when I first felt the lump;
You shared my fear.
You were there when they named it;
You shared my shock.
You were there when they took it;
You shared my loss.
You were there when I waited;
You shared my helplessness.
You were there for the prognosis;
You shared my relief.

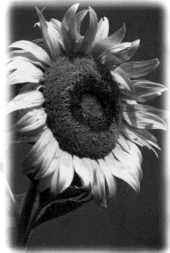

You were there when I weakened;
You strengthened me.
You were there when I cried;
You held me.
You were there when I raged;
You soothed me.
You were there when I doubted;
You believed in me.
You were there for the children;
When I couldn't be.

You've been at my side every step of the way,
And I love you.

Wednesday, October 29

An ordinary weekday, an ordinary routine…

#1 Take the girls to school.
#2 Go to work.
#3 Swim to keep the shoulder loose.
#4 Make a Halloween costume
…and so on.

Everyone thinks I have made a marvelous recovery. None of them realize I am just living by numbers.

JUXTAPOSITION

Waging war each morning with confusion and despair.
Forcing each step forward, trying not to think nor care.
Reaching with persistence for a normal day's routine.
Trying now to take my weight and not on others lean.

Exercising frantically to gain back some control.
Fighting off the feelings that are weighing down my soul.
Aching in my shoulder, sore from elbow up to chest.
Looking almost normal in a new prosthetic breast.

Learning how to live with odds that threaten future life.
Thanking friends and relatives whose love has eased the strife.
Comforting my children who've been acting out their fear.
Working with new clients and resuming my career.

Dreading all the treatment that still lies ahead of me.
Facing reconstruction as the price of symmetry.
Feeling slightly crazy in a schizophrenic way.
Keeping faith tomorrow's dawn will bring a better day.

Monday, November 3

I seem to be living an immense lie. I hope no one notices. The more I pretend to be back to normal, the more crazy I feel. Just surviving each day has become an enormous task.

TRICHOTOMY

How are you doing?

"Incredibly well," my appearance replies,
"With my silicone breast and increased exercise.
I'm able to laugh and converse with rapport.
Incredibly well...I'm the same as before!"

How are you doing?

"Disturbingly changed" is my body's refrain,
"With an arm that can't move without causing me pain
And an image that's altered, unbalanced at core.
Disturbingly changed...not the same as before!"

How are you doing?

"Unbearably lost" is my soul's dark report,
"With a sense of defeat from a battle unfought.
All emotions in turmoil, each waging a war.
Unbearably lost...to return nevermore!"

Wednesday, November 12

We spent last week in Canada. It was wonderful. I came back thinking I was restored to my old self, but it must have been an illusion.

CIRCLES

In conceit I'd believed I would heal
In a line straight and true,
From beginning to end.

I'd endure each sharp facet of pain
With such courage and faith,
That I'd quickly return to my norm.

But life doesn't relinquish controls to conceit,
And I find I have traveled a line
That is curved to a ring.

The end I'd perceived has the feel of the place I began,
And I find myself fighting old battles with feelings
I'd thought had been won.

Friday, December 5

The more steps I take towards recovery, the more I am faced with how I have been changed. The loneliness has become overpowering, for this is not a time that others find easy to understand. Their grief for my loss has run its course. Mine has much further to go.

DEPRESSION

"Prepare for depression," were words that they'd used.
I'd expected grey mists of despair,
Not this seething black force that compresses my soul
And consumes all ambition and care.

"Prepare for depression," they said once again.
Did they know I'd awaken each day
To a body so changed, the mind couldn't accept
Emotions its grief would betray.

I've found the depression, or it has found me.
I'm attempting to combat its might.
It's taking all strength from my body and soul,
And I'm frightened I'm losing the fight.

It freezes all actions without giving rest.
It suffocates feelings and hope.
It causes withdrawal of senses thus numbed
And relieves them of pressures to cope.

Is this the depression of which I was warned?
Is it here I'm expected to stay,
In the midst of this fight, in the bowels of despair,
As each ounce of my strength ebbs away?

I'm so lonely amidst all this darkness and loss.
But I mustn't allow it to win.
I must force myself forwards each difficult day
And allow those who love to come in.

I'll ignore the rejection of those who can't give
And accept the great love and support
That I find all around, when I trouble to look,
Hoping soon that the fight will be fought.

"Prepare for depression," words easy to say.
But the truth I've uncovered, with tears,
Is I could not prepare in advance for such hell,
But must battle it as it appears.

Tuesday, December 16

I have never been one of those people who grumbles about Christmas. I normally love every facet of it. But this year I do not feel like celebrating anything.

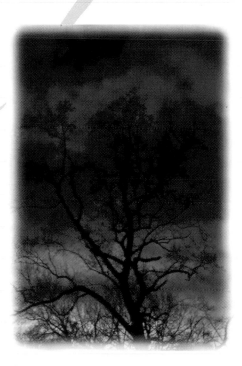

CHRISTMAS LOVE

Mum, give up! Give us the job!
We'll gladly trim the tree.
Don't fight the tears, just let them flow.
Allow yourself to be.
It's known as fact that Christmastime
Makes poignant any grief,
So let us take the painful jobs.
Let's give you some relief.

For several months we've been enraged.
You've not been at our side.
We didn't want to face the fact
Our mother might have died.
We didn't want to see you ill,
For all along we knew,
There's no one in this world of ours
Could take the place of you.

So while we've watched you fight despair
And struggle to reclaim
Your life and health, the way it was,
We've battled fear and shame.
Our dream was to provide support,
Take cancer in our stride.
We didn't manage very well,
But Mum, we always tried.

So sit and let us trim the tree,
You'll see how we prepare
For Christmas, as you've always taught.
Each detail will be there,
The cards and stockings hung in place,
The crèche with star above.
And then we'll add the final touch:
We'll fill the house with love.

Monday, December 29

The depression has been greatly eased by all of the love and support I have received over the holidays. I am feeling much better. I have even arranged to go skiing tomorrow.

SKI FREE

I'd forgotten my body could move
With such speed
Down a hill.

I'd forgotten my pulses could race
With this sense
Of pure thrill.

I'd forgotten the shock of the
Cold biting air
On my face.

I'd forgotten the feel of my heart
In my mouth
At such pace.

I'm in love with this sense
Of abandon,
This purified air.

I'm enmeshed in this world
Of fast motion, this world
Full of dare.

I'm renewed by a body
That skis, all day long,
Without rest.

I'm released for a while
From the burden of
Losing my breast.

PART TWO

RECONSTRUCTION

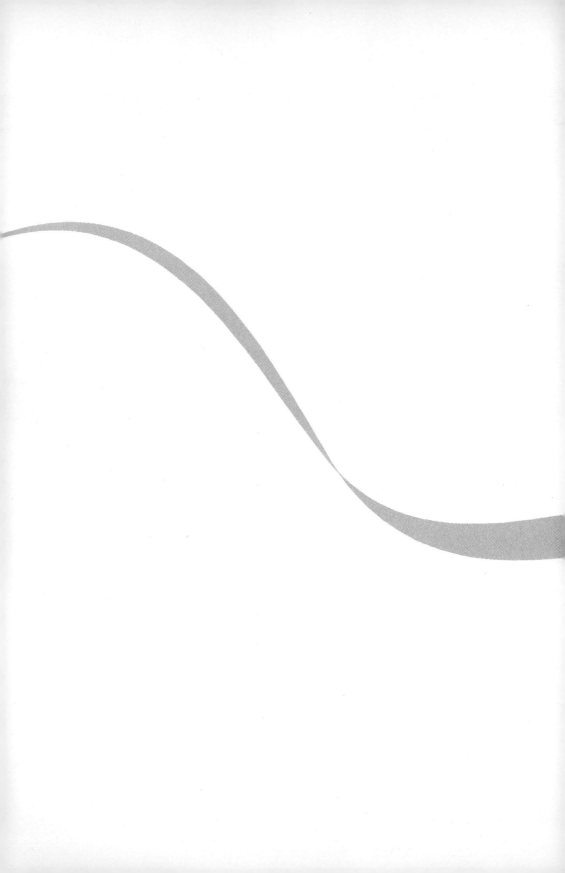

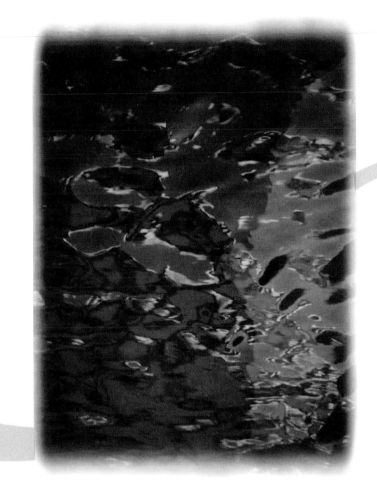

4 • A TIME FOR AMBIVALENCE

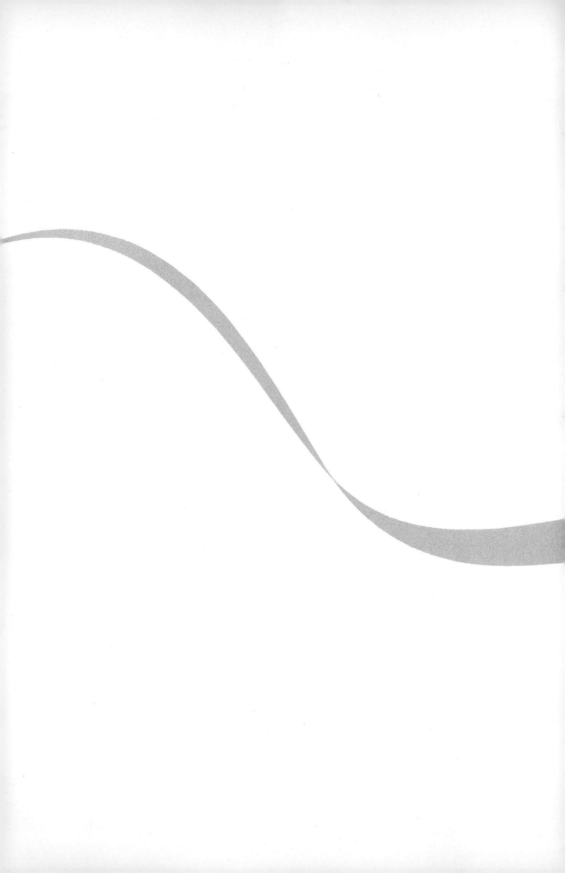

Thursday, January 1

Despite my newly achieved physical fitness, I feel incomplete. Subtle echoes of rape and disconnectedness remain deep within my soul. Final decisions about reconstruction hover perilously close over the horizon. Merely thinking about them is sending me into panic.

TIGHTROPE

Yet another silk thread, in a mist of fine dew,
Holds my spirit aloft lest it fall.
But my mind is bereft of all things it once knew,
And new fears have my soul in their thrall.

This path feels the same as the one months ago.
Though my head tells my heart of the lie,
I cannot believe that the terrors won't grow,
And I freeze with each step that I try.

Again nothing to do but continue to prove
I can walk down this thread so unsafe,
With ears shut against doubts that assail every move
And bereft of all senses but faith.

Saturday, January 3

I am in terrible pain about this decision. The guilt of putting myself and my family through more trauma is immense. Breast reconstruction seems to carry such a judgment.

VOICES

Mastectomy! Cancer!
How distressing! How young!
How shocking the loss!
How courageous! How strong!

Reconstructing a breast?
How eccentric! How vain!
How foolish the need!
How distasteful the pain!

We approved of your grief,
Tore our hair for your plight,
But we think you should see
That you can't make it right!

Perhaps it's your mate
Who is making the fuss,
For the loss of your breast
Has ceased hurting us.

In fact we're quite through
All the terror and pain.
We've managed it well,
We've no more to gain.

So we can't understand
Your insatiable need
To be whole once again.
It's insufferable greed.

If you go your own way
Through this tasteless affair,
Don't expect our support
Or continuing care.

Last time we faced death,
Waging heart-stopping war.
This time there is nothing
For us but a bore!

Monday, January 5

The surgery is confirmed for Friday. Again I am torn. The doctors have told me that even with the reconstruction, I will not feel symmetrical unless they alter the right breast to match the reconstructed side. I do not want them to touch it; it is the only one I have left.

SYMMETRY

Another day,
Another month,
Another year,
Another trip
To the hospital.

Another room,
Another nurse,
Another plan,
Another man
In a white coat.

Another bed,
Another shot,
Another sleep,
Another breast
Changed from its norm.

Another loss,
Another pain,
Another grief,
Another lack
Of easy choices.

Wednesday, January 7

I have agreed to let them alter the other breast. Only John seems to be able to understand my grief about this decision.

SO WHAT?

Uplift and tighten!
You ought to be glad.
You'll have a young look,
So why be so sad?

I liked the old look.
My breasts were just fine.
Let my daughters look younger,
I'm near thirty-nine!

Friday, January 9

Another D day. More than anything else, I
want to feel whole again. I want to be able to
hold my husband and children in my arms
without bumping their heads against my rib cage.
My time for ambivalence is over. I am resolved.

DEADLINE #2

For months I have struggled
To walk without looking ahead.
Large parts of my soul have been
Trapped in a mire of deep dread.

The grief of allowing myself
To be altered again by the knife
Was the feeling I'd known when
I gave up my breast for my life.

Today, as I pass once again
Through the surgical door,
My eyes are unveiled, and I see
That it's not like before.

Last time, all I felt was
Confusion, dark terror, and grief.
Today, I give thanks for my chance
At this step bringing future relief.

5 · A TIME FOR ADAPTATION

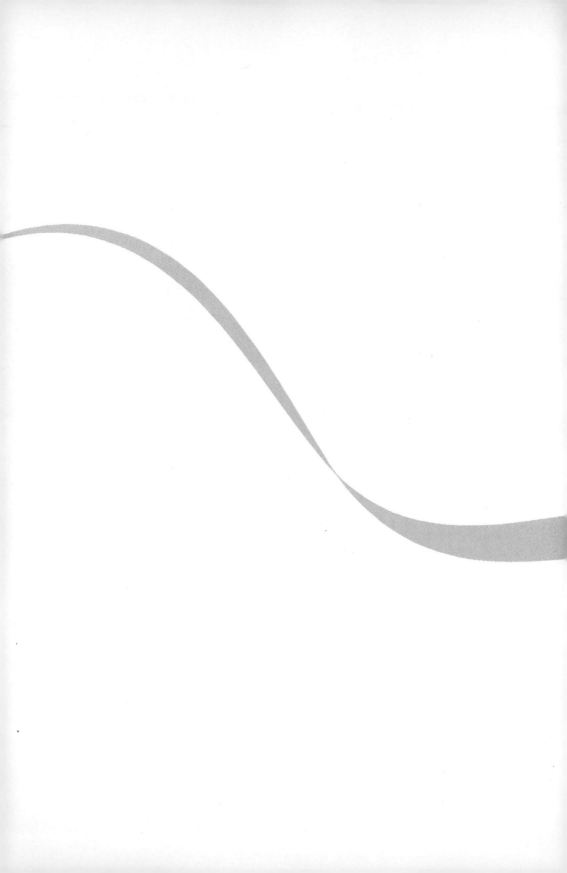

Saturday, January 10

If this is a postanesthetic high...I'll take a dozen. In the first instant of consciousness, my soul was aware of the difference in my body. Its missing piece had been restored.

WHOLE! WHOLE! WHOLE!

Let me shout!
Let me sing!
Let me strip!
Can you see?
I am whole!

I'm in pain.
I still mourn.
I still grieve.
I am changed,
But I am whole.

I fill space once again on each side.
Look! My spirit soars high in its pride.
Let me shout out my secret worldwide:

"I AM WHOLE!"

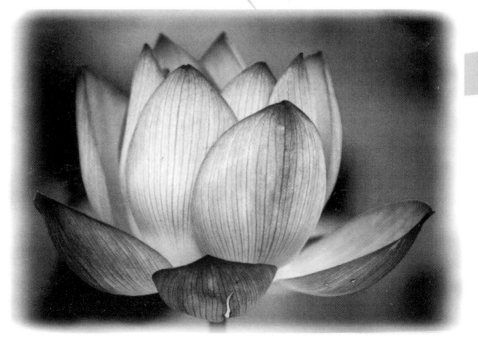

Sunday, January 11

They have just removed the dressings. I look great.

A BONUS...
THAT'S WHAT!

Tightened, uplifted,
Surprised to be glad.
They're right, I look younger.
I'm not at all sad.

Though I liked my old look,
My new breasts are just great.
Not young as in daughters'
But a young thirty-eight!

Tuesday, January 13

6.00 a.m....The honeymoon period is over. The nightmares have started again.

TRAPDOOR

Earthquakes and war; bombs explode in my head.
I awaken to terror, I am frozen with dread.
Night Goblins are out again casting their lure.
They're thrilled to discover my cancer trapdoor.

It's opened before several times in the day.
Its lock mechanism quite often gives way.
It responds to a word, or a look, or a tone,
And "Bang!" into fears about cancer I'm thrown.

It's worse though at night, when the Goblins like best
To hand out these nightmares to me as a test,
To see if I'll fall for their terror-filled dreams,
Thus open my soul to its own silent screams.

As blood stops its pounding and breath starts to flow,
I try to review all the things that I know.
I begin to accept the hard facts of this strife:
These fears about cancer are with me for life.

Tuesday, January 13

8.00 a.m....The surgeon who performed my mastectomy has just left the room. He dropped by for a visit and found me in terror from the nightmare. I am not even his patient at this time, and he must have had a hundred other things to do. He did not do them. He chose to stay with me and hold my hand until my terror abated and the trapdoor closed. His healing gift was that of time.

NEVER A NUMBER

I was never a number,
For you don't treat numbers...
Just people.
Each person is special
To you.

Your belief is that
Nothing is bad,
Only good...and then
Better.

You talked of a cup
Being full
Halfway up,
Or empty
Half down.

This was hard to accept,
For I had the cancer,
Not you.
But you didn't just heal,
You gave love
In its humblest form.

You knew you weren't God,
Put on this earth to heal man.
Just a human with skill
And an honest desire to be part of this fight
Against suffering and death,
With just human tools.

You gave me the truth from day one.
You answered each question
Again and again,
For I needed to ask them
Again and again.

No matter the rush,
You never rushed me,
Nor anyone else.

You allowed me my space in this fight.
You heard my concerns,
Allowed me to choose,
Then supported the choice.
With a sense of respect and of worth,
You encouraged my efforts to heal.

You gave me your hand.
You gave me your care.
You gave me your skills.
You gave me your prayers.

I gave you my hand.
I gave you my fears.
I gave you my trust.
I gave you my truth.
I made a commitment to heal.

We have shared the same journey
From a different approach.
We've both grown, we've both learned,
And slowly...
I heal.

Monday, January 19

I have just heard that my job security is being threatened. How can the bottom of my life keep falling out in this way?

CONFUSION

Gently depressed,
But quite unaware
Of its cause.

Too weary to fight;
Lost, alone,
Amidst echoes of wars.

Relieved with great joy
By a body restored
To its whole.

Shocked by the damage
Past onslaughts have wrought
To the soul.

Troubled by costs
Reduced income must
Struggle to bear.

Frightened by news
That my job may
No longer be there.

Confused by the thought
I must somehow
Deserve all this strife.

Reprieved by the truth:
There's a time for all things
In one's life.

Weakened by doubts
As I question
What next year will bring.

Strengthened by Nature's
Great hope, as she
Heralds in Spring.

Loved well by those
Who've supported each step
Of the way.

Grateful for life and its gifts
Every hour
Of each day.

Saturday, January 24

They have started to expand the temporary implant. I will be glad when the final one is permanently in place. My body is becoming increasingly confused by the constant changes.

SHIFTING IMAGES

In four months I've been changed
To the point I now doubt who I am.
First, from woman I moved
To a guise that portrayed half a man.
I've been changed once again,
Back to whole, but my head's in a whirl,
For this time I was changed from half man
Back to woman, with curves of a girl.

For some reason it's hard
To adapt to this body renewed.
I'm completely restored;
I am also intangibly skewed.
I am tired of this road.
It's too long, and of grief I'd be free.
But I can't seem to hurry my soul
To accept this new image of me.

Monday, January 26

The confusion is getting worse. I have started to take consolation in food.

WILD-GOOSE CHASE

Compulsively eating,
As if that will help me renew
My acquaintance with self.

Will it help to establish control
Over boundaries changed?

I remember this need came before,
After losing the breast.
Only then I had desperately sought
To replace what was lost.

It is now, as it was at that time,
A futile attempt
Of a subconscious will
To recoup its old form.

Destined to fail,
Lost from the start,
Gaining with all of its force,
Only weight.

Wednesday, January 28

This winter seems to be endless. The world lies trapped under a blanket of snow. It suffers in silence. Would that I could do likewise.

IRRITATION

Impatient with feelings
That block my straight road
Up ahead,

I'd thought a path cleared.
But I face new frustration
Instead.

When I found myself whole,
I'd believed that the end was
In sight.

Yet more feelings intrude,
Causing chaos and slowing
The fight.

I'm so ready to heal,
I can smell the sweet scent
Of success.

But I'm forced to take time
Sorting feelings
I'd rather repress.

I can see where to go.
I just wish there were some
Other way.

I'm so bored with myself
And fed up of each
Step-by-step day.

Monday, February 2

I had assumed that if I regained my sense of being whole, I would feel integrated. I was wrong.

TRICHOTOMY #2

How are you doing?

"Altered, indeed," my appearance replies,
"I've a nippleless breast that's lopsided in size.
The silicone breast, I can't use anymore.
Altered, indeed…Not the same as before."

How are you doing?

"A little bit odd," is my body's refrain,
"I flinch now and then with occasional pain.
The implant feels strange, but I'm balanced at core.
A little bit odd…But improved from before."

How are you doing?

"Completely restored," is my soul's great report,
"The victory's mine, the battle's cut short.
I don't sense my looks changed, I don't care that I'm sore.
I'm completely restored…to the same as before."

Wednesday, February 4

5.00 a.m....I could not sleep, I am so excited. I have survived this thirty-ninth year!

CELEBRATIONS

It's a red-letter day.
Bring out candles and cake.
Bring out hats and balloons,
A great party we'll make.
A glass of fine wine,
Let's give toast to the year.
It's a red-letter day...
For my birthday is here.

On no birthday before
Have I been so aware
Of each minute fulfilled,
Of each breath of fresh air.
For each friend, for each child
For my husband so dear,
I give thanks from my heart,
Now my birthday is here.

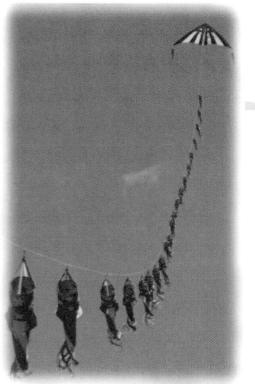

In the thirty-eight past
There's been none like today.
Not one brought the urge
To shout loud, "Hip hooray,"
To jump high with joy
And with gratitude cheer,
"Let's celebrate life
Through my fortieth year!"

Thursday, February 12

The final surgery is tomorrow. The temporary implant will be replaced by a permanent one, and the nipple will be reconstructed. It is supposed to be less involved than the previous surgeries. I have been awaiting this day for weeks. I cannot understand why, deep down, I am feeling so desperate.

HIDDEN RAGE

The panic's rising, doubts abound, the final day draws near.
Instead of joy at this event, I find I'm trapped by fear.
I doubt that I can stand more pain, I doubt I'll like my breast.
I'm frightened that when all is done I'll fail this final test.

I want to be the way I was before the cancer came,
And even though the breast looks good, it's nothing like the same.
I've tried to hide these doubts and fears, I've told myself, "Behave!"
I've tried to count my blessings when I've seen what others brave.

But now I find if I'm to heal, I must reject this sham.
No matter who I want to be, I'm left with who I am.
I must allow all good and bad to integrate and flow,
For when I keep them far apart, I find I cannot grow.

It's hard to open up my soul to truths that I've denied.
It makes me feel pathetic, lost…a whiner lacking pride.
But as defenses crumble down, I face the war I wage.
Deep down inside, the truth's revealed in tidal waves of rage.

I'm mad as hell the cancer came. I'm mad that it chose me.
Enraged to have to mourn my breast, enraged to not be free.
Enraged I've lost my innocence and faith in life ahead.
Enraged that all my dreams and plans are faintly tinged with dread.

I'm left within this wake of rage, a little sad and drained,
But find by pushing through denial a greater wisdom's gained.
The cancer is the cause of all my buried rage and grief,
Not this new breast, whose only aim is to provide relief.

Though not completely perfect, this new breast can restore
My sense of being whole again, full female at my core.
It cannot take the pain away, it cannot stop the rage.
But it can help to soften both as I move through this stage.

Illusions of a final phase thus gently disappear.
The pain from feelings unresolved disproves the end is near.
But as I let these feelings hurt, their presence not denied,
I've faith that, though this route is tough, I'm healing from inside.

Saturday, February 28

    This has been a hard two weeks. I was sick after the anesthetic, and now I have developed another severe urinary tract infection.

A QUESTION OF TIME

How long will it be
'Til my body is mine
Once again?
How long before
Forceps, bright needles,
Sharp scalpels, and sutures
Are through?
How long before I can regain
A figure whose shape stays the same,
A body that's free from all pain?
How long?

How long will it be
'Til I'm no longer
Weary and worn?
How long before
Nightmares of terrors
Or hours without sleeping
Are done?
How long 'til my eyes can accept
Without tears what the mirrors reflect,
Viewing life once again with respect?
How long?

Monday, March 2

Today, I looked in the mirror and burst into tears.

ADAPTATION

The wrong shape,
The wrong size,
The nipple's too far to the side.

I'm sure that it's slipping
And stitches are
Breaking inside.

I don't like this new look,
Though my family and friends say
It's fine.

I don't know this new breast,
So I'm sure that it cannot
Be mine.

My breast filled a space in
A manner completely
Its own.

I'd had it from birth,
And each part of its growth
I had known.

When I lost it, I cried,
But believed in my
Innermost soul,

Reconstructing the breast
Would replace it and
Make me feel whole.

It has made me feel whole.
Nonetheless, there's still
Grief to be borne,

For no breast, even new,
Could replace one...
So loved and well worn!

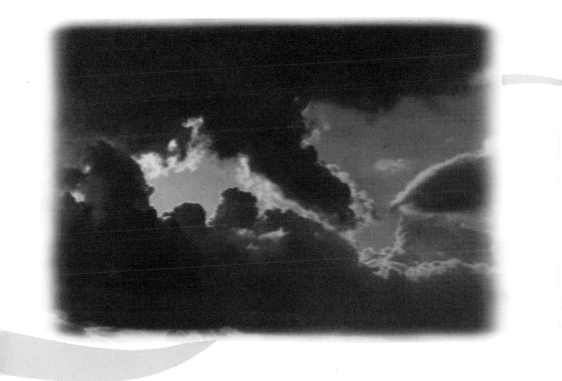

6 · A TIME FOR TANGENTS

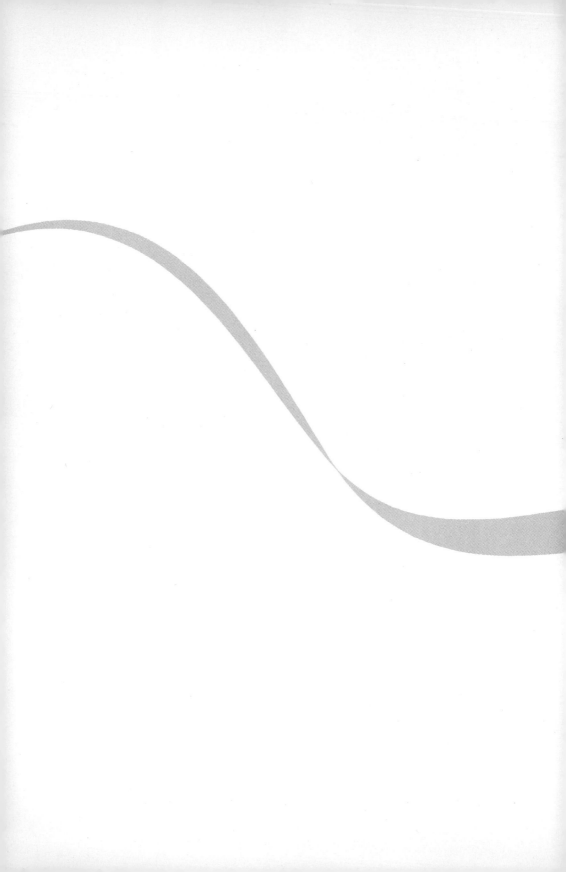

Tuesday, March 24

Two weeks ago I had a mammogram on my other breast. The results were questionable. Yesterday, the sonogram was clearer. It showed abnormal tissue that may prove to be more cancer. A biopsy is scheduled for April 2.

THE OTHER SIDE OF FEAR

I never understood before
How special was each hour,
How smallest seconds of my time
Were endless in their power
To fill my life with beauty, peace,
With joy in simple things.
I never understood before
How much each second brings.

I never understood before
The love surrounding me,
Its depth, its warmth, its healing force,
Its gift completely free,
Its power throughout the darkest times
To penetrate despair.
I never understood before
How much most people care.

I never understood before
The beauty of this world,
How tiny petals of each plant
Were miracles unfurled,
How birds could fill the skies with song,
How webs were touched by dew.
I never understood before,
This world I thought I knew.

I never understood before
The strength within my soul,
How it could help my anxious mind
Develop new control,
How it could calm my troubled nights
And make all things more clear.
I never understood before
The other side of fear.

Thursday, April 30

The biopsy showed no malignancies. Unfortunately, I had no time to rejoice in the news: on the day they removed the sutures, I suffered the most vicious urinary tract infection to date. The doctors do not think these recurrent infections are from cancer, but they cannot be sure. I am scheduled for a cystoscopy on May 5. I could scream!

OVERLOAD

Too much to handle
In too short a time.
ENOUGH!

Lost amidst attitudes
Smugly sublime.
ALONE!

Bounced between doctors
With all different aims.
SPLIT UP!

Few comprehending how
Each treatment maims.
DETACHED!

Greeted by folks who
Are bored by my plight.
TOO LONG!

Fear in their eyes
For an unending fight.
REPELLED!

Each new attack
Draining efforts to cope.
WORN OUT!

Witnessing slowly
Erosion of hope.
DESPAIR!

Sunday, May 3

I have made an appointment to go for counseling. It is time to ask for help.

MARKED TRAILS

Fifty minutes of space
Where it's safe to unload
All the burdens I bear.

Fifty minutes of time
To explore, without judgment,
My darkest despair.

Fifty minutes of freedom
To whine, without caring
What others will say.

Fifty minutes of guidance
And help, with a nudge
When I try to delay.

Fifty minutes reviewing
The past, with each facet
That's part of the whole.

Fifty minutes acknowledging
Pain that is common
To everyone's soul.

Fifty minutes accepting
Events which have led
To these difficult days.

Fifty minutes exploring
Life's gifts, with attempts
To discover new ways.

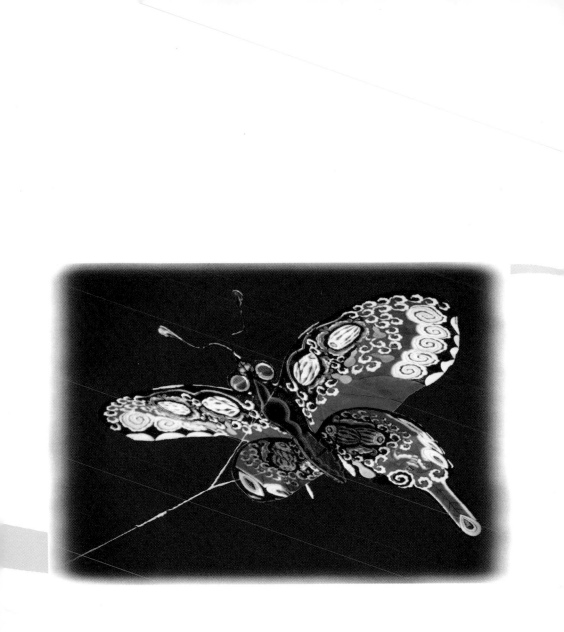

7 · A TIME FOR REINTEGRATION

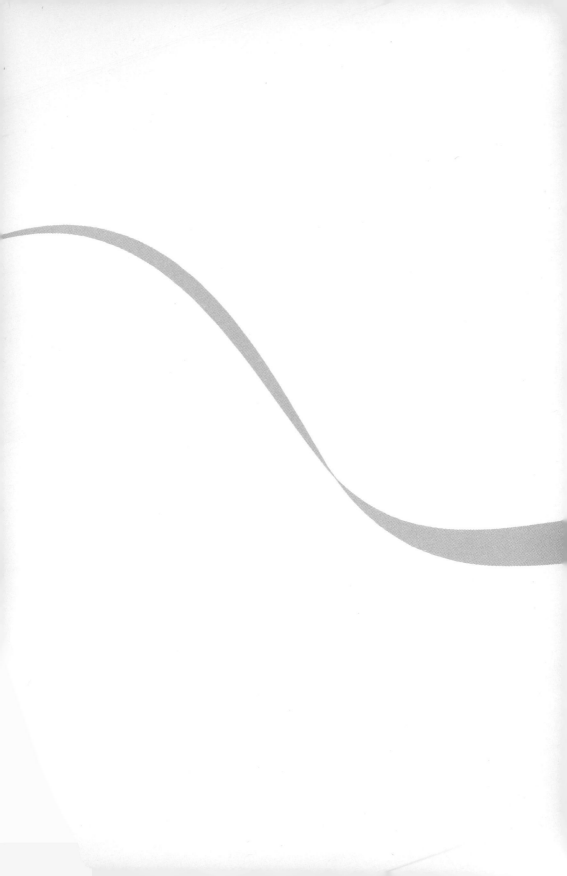

Thursday, May 14

The reconstruction is now healed, and it is looking good. The tests have shown no cancer, and the despair has lifted. I feel that I should be forging ahead. Instead, I seem to be stuck.

NO-MAN'S-LAND

A strange sterile place between sickness and health,
A void that is empty of air,
A stillness of soul that's had too little choice,
Whose substance seems sapped of all care.

A strange sterile stand on a fine-balanced scale,
At a point between fate and control,
Where the need to move on in the struggle to heal
Is weighed 'gainst the victim's safe role.

A strange sterile peace in the eye of the storm,
With no need to defend or attack,
With no Jesters of Fate to create further stress...
Thus no will, if there were, to fight back.

A strange sterile time, but a time that must change,
A time bringing rest and respite,
A time to digest all the onslaught before,
And a time to prepare a new fight.

Friday, May 22

The counseling has continued to help me enormously, and I seem to be moving forward once again. Yet I am still strangely out of sync with my surroundings. I cannot stop talking about myself, even to those whom I have just met. Most people have been generous in their acceptance of this. Others have not.

A MIXED MESSAGE

What a lovely swimsuit, your figure's so trim.
I've watched you each day from afar.
As you've swam all those lengths, I've envied your youth
And your health....No, I've noticed no scar.

I withdraw as I hear of your past awful months,
For I find if I try to relate
All that pain within one who is so full of life,
I am faced by my own mortal state.

So you'll have to forgive my cool nod as we pass,
For the fact is, I don't wish to see
The real truth that's between every line of your tale.
For that truth is...it could have been me.

Tuesday, June 16

I am becoming secure enough to start keeping my own counsel. However, it is no easier to meet new people. It is as if I have lost myself in the past year's confusion. I no longer seem to know who I am.

DISSONANCE

Hello, pleased to meet you.
I wish you could see
The panic concealed
Behind self-assured me.
I'm not as I was
In the years gone before.
In some ways I am less,
Though, in some, I'm much more.

Hello, pleased to meet you.
You'd think I were strange
If I'd tried to impart
How I'm coping with change,
How this body before you,
Though healthy and whole,
Feels three months in age
'Round a forty-year soul.

There's no room as we meet
For these factors to share.
There's no room in small talk
For my soul to lay bare.
Thus, I'm forced to present
A most confident sham
Of the person I was,
Not the one I now am.

So though pleased to meet you,
I'm thrown into pain
By these roles I act out,
By these fronts I maintain.
For deep in my soul
Hidden voices insist
This person you're meeting
Has ceased to exist.

Saturday, July 11

During the past few months, I have noticed how the largest difficulties often took their origins from the smallest sources. Some of the toughest times were caused by a casual opening social gambit of "How are you?" I never knew how to reply. The truth was unacceptable, and the lie was hard to give. What joy I experienced today when, with equanimity and truth, I was able to reply, "Fine."

TRICHOTOMY RESOLVED

How are you doing?

"At peace with the change" my appearance replies,
"My shape is now normal to discerning eyes.
The scars that I bear show I've been through the wars.
At peace with the change...again safe on home shores."

How are you doing?

"Altered but healed" is my body's refrain,
"Slight losses in strength, slight discomforts remain.
My lovemaking's changed, but intense as before.
I'm altered but healed...well adapted at core."

How are you doing?

"Rejoicing in life" is my soul's new report,
"Embracing the future with skills the past taught.
Infused with new growth, now an integral whole,
Reunited as one are...mind, body, and soul!"

Sunday, July 12

At last I can say, without reservation, that the reconstruction was worth all of the ambivalence and adaptation. Once again, I discovered the most difficult times were eased by the compassionate care and affection of yet another unusual surgeon.

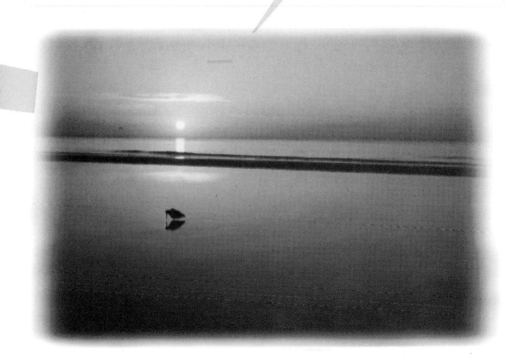

A MAN OF DEEP FEELINGS

A man of deep feelings,
Ensconced behind natural reserve,
You reached through my pain.
One hug gave me faith to endure
That most difficult day.

I faltered in fear,
And you waited.
I faltered again.
You stood still,
Always giving me time,
So much time.

You basked in my joy
At again being whole.
You stood ground,
Never turning away,
When I found the new breast
Was no longer the one
I had lost.

You offered your skills
With a burning desire
To replace, re-create,
Always seared by the truth
You could never undo
What was done,
Always giving your best
And allowing me time
To give mine.

You provided a shelter,
Allowing me freedom
To search for a truth
Which you knew,
And which I finally learned:
Reconstruction is not restoration,
Reconstruction helps reintegration.

Wednesday, July 15

My successful return to health is now a fact. I am back to normal. Everyone is noticing the difference. At last I am ready to reconnect with my world.

MATURING WORLDS

Where is the world I left behind?
That's what I'd like to know,
Where children play in innocence
Where fields of flowers grow,
Where nature's joy pervades the air
With scents and sounds so clear.
Where is the world I left behind,
The one that knows no fear?

Where is the world I left behind?
I must have lost my way.
For I've returned from journeys far,
To find with great dismay
A world that's full of swamps and mists,
With stumps of rotting trees,
And nothing in the silent air,
Not even Nature's breeze.

Where is the world I left behind?
It can't be this one here.
For I have paid my price in pain
And suffering and fear.
And I believed if I endured,
To pass the final test,
I'd have my old world back again,
Where safely I could rest.

But now I see that's not to be.
My old world's left behind,
And if I want to live life full,
I'd better try to find
Some substance in the world that's here,
The secrets of its pain,
Its older sense of harmony,
Its more mature refrain.

As slowly I accept this world,
Embrace it as my own,
I find that next to stumps and swamps
Old forest glades have grown.
And Nature's peace has filled the air
That's heavy with a dew.
And now I see this world has more
Than that which I once knew.

For this world is an old, old world.
It bears what can't be borne.
It nurtures weary travelers,
Arriving frayed and worn.
It sings a song of life from death
And has a place for both.
This world has known the pain of man
And witnessed all his growth.

And thus it came to be my world
When I faced death and strife,
By sacrificing innocence
To harsher truths of life.
At last I see the world I left.
It rests where it should be,
At peace beside more youthful worlds
In cherished memory.

Friday, August 7

As I look around, I see that my world has not been the only one to change. The safe worlds of my children . . . Kelly aged 19, Erin aged 17, and Samantha aged 11 . . . have also been altered. During the past year, each of them has faced terror, and each in her own way has grown through it.

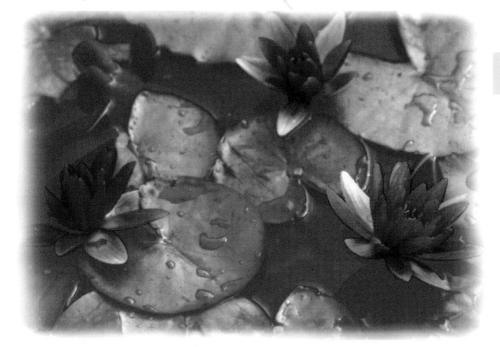

TRIPLE BLESSING

ERIN...
Child of my mind,
Who guided me time and again
Through the fire.
The child who could not look away
From my pain
And so suffered with me.
The child who so wanted to run
From it all,
But who still stood her ground,
In terror and pain,
With eyes closed and teeth bared,
Never slacking her grip
On her love for me.

SAMANTHA...
Child of my soul,
Who so valiantly sought
        to discover
Some sense in it all.
The child whose unquenchable
Zest for all life
Infused hope,
Through those darkest of days.
The child who
        so steadfastly fought
Her despair
And then tackled mine,
In confusion and doubt,
But determined to win,
Never letting my soul turn away
From the living of life.

KELLY...
Child of my heart,
Whose distance
        from home gave
A sense of unreal
To it all.
The child who
        so battled her urge
To ignore all the pain,
Lest it make her unsafe.
The child who need not
        have come home,
But who did,
Every chance that she had.
Frozen with fear,
Numbed at her core,
Not daring to reach out
        and touch,
She stayed by my side.

Thursday, August 20

The summer is passing. It has been a good one. I am discovering that many things are better for nearly having lost them.

JOY IN THE AIR

Is the air smelling sweeter?
Or is it the way that I feel
As I lie on the beach
And bask in the sun
Without shame,
In my well-loved bikini,
The one I had feared
I would not need again?

Is the wind blowing fresher?
Or is it the frame of my mind
As I splash in the waves
At my children and mate,
And get splashed in return
As the play escalates,
While loud shrieks of excitement
And laughter resound?

Wednesday, September 2

Another anniversary. It is a year to the day since I had that first mammogram. I am due for another one next week. I am also due for my routine annual bone scan, chest X ray, and blood test. These examinations and their accompanying anxiety are becoming a small, but necessary, part of my life, for I have had cancer.

CONNECTING LINES

The same mothers and children
In line for their books
As last Fall.
The same school,
The same scents in the air.
I breathe...and flash back
To the dread and confusion
I'd felt the last time
In this line,
When I'd chattered and smiled
And had wondered,
"Would I be alive,
Or would there be space
In my place
In this line
The next time?"

I don't think of these things
Very much
Anymore.
Just a flicker of thought
Now and then.
For I'm cured,
More or less.
Though no one knows which
Quite for sure.
So I live for the hour,
I plan for the year,
I hope for the best...
And I pray,
In my way,
Every day.

Saturday, September 19

The mammogram was normal. I am now freed from tests for another twelve months. Last year on this date, in shock and terror, I faced my mastectomy and its results. Today I rejoice in my recovered health. My time for healing is nearly over. As I look back on this year, I can see that my journey through trauma has also brought gifts and blessings. These are now mine to inherit.

NEW DIMENSIONS

I'm aware that my soul has gained strength
From the blessings received.
I've developed new faith in old concepts
I'd never believed.
I have found I am loved for myself,
Not the things that I do.
I have learned how to live for the day,
Counting blessings anew.

I've accepted there's things in my life
That I cannot control.
I've encountered ill health, fear, and loss
From the patient's hard role.
I've gained insights from this and results
That I couldn't foretell.
I have found that in order to heal
I don't need to be well.

I'm amazed I'm restored to the point
I confuse the left side.
I'm entranced by the fact I can wear
Even swimsuits with pride.
I am thankful for medical help
And the care I've received.
For I'm whole once again,
And my life's been reprieved.

I've explored newfound skills to facilitate
Tension release.
I've acquired deeper wisdom, through chaos,
A new inner peace.
I have witnessed the love of my family
And friends, all so dear.
I have come to love life even more
Through the pain of this year.

Finally...

One in every eight women in the United States develops breast cancer as she ages. However, the actual experience of coping with it is a very individual one. There are many common feelings and concerns, and I gained great relief from talking to others who had traveled a similar road.

THE CHAIN

Cynthia...
So quietly brave,
You reached out to touch
My despair.
So different from me,
With a strength firmly rooted
In prayer.
You shared my deep loss
And encouraged my
Efforts to heal.
Your own battles with cancer,
You selflessly tried
To conceal.

Sally...
Bouncing with life,
A stranger, you came
To my side.
You showed me your scars
And new breast with
Great joy and such pride.
You shared your hard journey,
You hoped you'd remain
Cancer free.
I rail at the Fates
That refused to permit this
To be.

Joanne...
Freed now from cancer,
But ready to help me
By phone.
You answered my questions,
Allaying my fears
By your tone.
Describing your journey
Through surgical steps
Up ahead,
You gave me the strength
To continue and lessened
My dread.

Sharon...
You're now taking steps
From the place where I stood
Months ago.
You've discovered the lump,
But results of the tests
You don't know.
I'm with you in thought,
As those women who shared
In my plight,
In the hope you'll gain strength
From our chain, as you start
Your own fight.